WEIGHT WATCHERS

77 DELICIOUS WEIGHT WATCHERS

RECIPES FOR RAPID WEIGHT LOSS!

By Sarah Lynch

The PointsPlus® and SmartPoints™ values for recipes are calculated by Sarah Lynch and are not an endorsement or approval of the product, recipe or its manufacturer or developer by Weight Watchers International, Inc., the owner of the PointsPlus® registered trademark and SmartPoints™ trademark.

Introduction

I want to thank you and congratulate you for downloading the book, Weight Watchers: 77 Delicious Weight Watchers Recipes For Rapid Weight Loss!

This book contains proven steps and strategies on how to why the Weight Watchers plan is best for a nutritional food program. It is chock-full of enticing, easy recipes that follow the Smart Points plan, many are even crock-pot dump recipes so that you can eat properly with a busy weekday schedule.

Weight Watchers encourages a lifestyle change, not a temporary fix to your weight dilemma. Choosing a healthy eating plan will enhance your energy and invigorate your health. When you follow their suggestions for meals and snacks, eating at the proper times with the suggested portions, you will achieve your weight loss goals.

Thanks again for downloading this book, I hope you enjoy it!

TABLE OF CONTENTS

Introduction

Chapter 1: Why Weight Watchers?

Chapter 2: How To Stay Motivated Losing Weight

Chapter 3: The Basics of Good Eating

Chapter: 4 Breakfast Recipes

Chapter 5: Soup and Salad Recipes

Chapter 6: Appetizers and Main Dishes

Chapter 7: Delicious Desserts

Chapter 8: Recipes With Zero Smart Points!

Chapter 9: Snacks With Only 1 Smart Point

Chapter 10: Snacks That Are Ready-Made With Only 4 or Less Smart Points!

Conclusion

CHAPTER 1: WHY WEIGHT WATCHERS?

Weight Watchers was designed by Jean Nidetch in the early 1960's, so it is not a new, fad diet. It has a proven success record for over fifty years, with thousands of testimonials from men and women like you. People who are stressed but very concerned about their weight. People that want to lose but don't want a lot of hassle figuring out the rules of the program.

The beauty of Weight Watchers is that it is customized for you, with no excluded foods, no weird food combinations, and no chemically laced additives. Weight Watchers is designed for the busy individual that is concerned with their weight and the health-giving quality of their food choices.

Weight Watchers is all about healthy portions and fresh foods, fruits and vegetables that boost your nutrition and satisfy your hunger. Weight Watchers emphasizes lifestyle changes, not just what you eat, but when you eat, how much you eat, plus the addition of exercise to keep your body moving strong.

Losing weight is a difficult endeavor. Most diet plans either exclude specific foods, which can be unhealthy and lead to organ failure, or limit your foods to only one thing, like a protein shake, which sets you up for failure when you have lost your weight. How will you handle the transition back to a normal diet? Most people can't and gain back all the weight loss and even more!

Weight Watchers helps you control your eating habits by utilizing Smart Points. Smart Points rewards you with weight loss when you eat the specified quantity that has been allocated only for you, according to your body weight and height, gender and age. It provides a customized number that gives you a daily allotment of points, plus a weekly allowance of splurges. There is even a special consideration for those "date nights" or eating out with friends, when you go to a restaurant and need to know how to order.

Smart Points are what this book is about, a collection of Weight Watchers recipes that expand your tastes while teaching you proper nutrition. Weight Watchers has a food plan that is chock full of delicious, nutritious, satisfying recipes that boosts your metabolism and provides the needed vitamins and minerals your body is craving.

Best of all is the nutritional education you will receive when you attend weight watcher meetings. A balanced diet is the only way to receive all the necessary vitamins, minerals, proteins and carbohydrates that are needed to maintain a healthy body. When you follow the Weight Watchers plan, you will find a new energy and vitality that comes from maintaining a healthy diet, combined with the needed exercise your body requires to function properly.

Chapter 2: How To Stay Motivated Losing Weight

Staying motivated when it comes to weight loss and fitness exercise can sometimes become so tough you may feel like giving up. Especially if you are having difficult time achieving your goal. Note that losing weight is a slow process and it takes total devotion to achieve it, this means that the key to getting rid of that weight and sticking to that diet is not about what you eat or the amount of exercise you do but your attitude towards this goal. It is necessary to stay motivated and not give up before you reach your goal.

The following tips will teach you how to stay motivated

Write down your reasons for wanting to lose that weight

This is really important and as well as the number one thing that will help you get motivated. Get a paper and write down some of the reason you want to lose your weight and why you need to stay on diet. Is it because you want to improve your physical status? Is it because you want to reduce your health risk? Maybe you want to be able to pull off your cloth or wear bikini in front of your friend and feel comfortable about your body. These questions will help you stay focus on why you start your diet in the first place. Place this paper where it is accessible to you, read through it every day or every week and you will be surprise how this will help.

Get supportive partners

Working out and staying diet on your own can become frustrating, but having a partner or joining some group who share similar goal will be of great help. Check in on your partner or one of your group member through phone call, email, or even visit him or her. Discuss some challenges you are facing about your diets and share ideas, help each other to stay motivated by going to the gym together or some healthy cooking class, have meetings with others with similar goals and learn new ideas. Getting involved in this support system will help you reach your goal.

Challenge yourself

There are lots of way you can challenge yourself. Doing little competition among your support group is one way to do it, do extra push, get competitive with your friends will go a long way to achieving your goal. Set a task for yourself, be it a particular exercise or sticking to a particular diet and work towards it. Tell yourself you can do it!

Reward yourself

Always reward yourself after achieving some of your set objectives or after losing a few pounds or meet a healthy meal goal. Find a reward system that is best for you. You can take a day or two days break to reward yourself, you can also buy yourself new workout material. Don't deny yourself of appreciating and celebrating your success. You will be surprise how this will motivate you.

Make your pet a workout buddy

Your cute dog is an alternative way you can have fun and workout at the same time. Take your dog on a walk a couple of meters or around the block. You can even play a fetch and catch game with the dog. This companion can also help you exercise your body and add to achieving your goal.

Surround yourself with positive materials

Stock your refrigerator and freezer with healthy food. Get rid of cookies, cake and ice cream stored in your cabinet. Decorate your dining with fruits and vegetables, mind what you eat and how you eat them. Make your workout materials accessible, don't leave them under a pile of used clothes. Arrange your environment to reflect your goal and you will find it easy to stay focus.

Get help from your Smartphone

There are lots of app available to your Smartphone that can help you set up a workout routine, get you motivated and teach you new ideas. Download some healthy eating app that will teach you some of the recipes to add to your weekly meal and help you stay on diet.

Decline constant check on your scale

As much as scale equipment will help you monitor your progress frequent, use of the scale can undermine your spirit and kill your motivation. Weighing yourself daily to help maintain your weight is not applicable when you are trying to lose weight as this may cause you some discouragement. For better track of your progress try checking your weight once a week or once in two weeks.

CHAPTER 3: THE BASICS OF GOOD EATING

A balanced diet is the optimal way for a person to take care of their body. If you want to be healthy, your diet should consist of fruits, dairy products, whole grain foods, vegetables in all colors, protein and water, tea and coffee. Elimination of even one of these foods without a healthy substitute will cause eventual vitamin and mineral loss that will cause physical symptoms and possible organ failure.

Hydration is just as important as eating the right foods. Water, 8 glasses, are necessary for your kidneys to work properly. The addition of tea and coffee are for your pleasure, but they do not substitute for water. Water is needed by the body to flush out the toxins and poisons that accumulate as waste.

One of the singular advantages of following the Weight Watchers diet is the consistent and safe weight loss. By following their plan of eating 3 meals a day and two or three snacks, you will be giving your body the adequate nutrition without either skipping meals or overindulging.

While you are giving your body a nutritional boost through providing it healthy foods, you will be increasing your daily exercise. Your goal will be to gradually increase your movement until you reach 30 minutes of exercise 5 times a week. The exercise regimen, along with the proper nutrition, should provide you with a steady weight loss of about 2 pounds a week.

What will be your specific results? You won't know until you aggressively follow the Weight Watchers food plan, combined with the exercise program. We DO know that you will feel much better, that your self esteem will grow, that you will have a new spring in your step, and that you will be a much healthier YOU!

The new healthy YOU is the best part, a gift for everyone is the blessing of good health.

CHAPTER: 4 BREAKFAST RECIPES

Now that you know about the weight watchers diet lets dive into some delicious breakfast recipes that have the number of Smart Points labeled with each one

Apple Maple Oatmeal in the Crockpot

1/4th of recipe (about 1 1/4 cups): 262 calories, 6g total fat (0.5g sat fat), 247mg sodium, 41.5g carbs, 9.5g fiber, 7.5g sugars, 12.5g protein -- Smart Points value : 6

Ingredients:

- 1/3 cup plain protein powder with about 100 calories per serving 2 cups unsweetened vanilla almond milk

- 2 cups chopped Fuji or Gala apples

- 1 cup steel-cut oats

- 5 packets no-calorie sweetener (like Truvia)

- 1 1/2 tbsp. chia seeds

- 2 tsp. cinnamon

- 2 tsp. maple extract 1/2 tsp. vanilla extract 1/4 tsp. salt

Directions:

Spray a crock pot with nonstick spray. Add the protein powder and 2 cups of hot water to the crock pot. Stir until evenly textured. All the rest of the ingredients, still until smooth. Cover and cook 8 hours on Low. Serve. Makes 4 servings.

Avocado Toast with Egg

Servings: 1 • Size: 1 toast • Smart Points: 6

Calories: 229 • Fat: 10 g • Carb: 23 g • Fiber: 5 g • Protein: 12 g • Sugar: 4 g Sodium: 223 mg • Cholesterol: 186 mg

Ingredients:

- 1 slice whole grain bread, toasted (1.5 oz)
- 1 oz mashed (1/4 small) avocado
- 1 large egg
- kosher salt and black pepper to taste

Directions:

Peel and smash the avocado in a bow with a fork. Salt and pepper to taste. Spray a nonstick skillet with cooking spray and cook the egg to your preference. Place the avocado on the toast, top with the cooked egg, and add salsa if desired.

Baked Egg Muffin Omelets All the Way

Servings: 6 • Size: 2 omelets • Smart Points: 4

Calories: 148 • Fat: 9 g • Carb: 3 g • Fiber: 0 g • Protein: 14 g Sugar: 0 g • Sodium: 287 mg • Cholesterol: 196 mg

Ingredients:

- 6 large whole eggs

- 6 large egg whites salt and black pepper

- 3 strips cooked chopped bacon

- 3 tablespoons thawed frozen spinach, drained, or fresh, chopped spinach 3 tbsp diced tomatoes

- 3 tbsp diced onion

- 3 tbsp cup diced bell pepper

- 2 oz shredded cheddar

Directions:

Set the oven for 350F and preheat. Grease the muffin tin with cooking spray. Whisk the eggs and egg whites together, then season with salt and pepper. Fold in the remaining ingredients. Bake 25 minutes until eggs are set. Makes 12 muffins.

Baked Oatmeal with Fruit and Nuts

Servings: 6 • Serving Size: 1/6th • Smart Points : 6

Calories: 211.7 • Fat: 5.4 g • Protein: 5.6 g • Carb: 38.1 g • Fiber: 3.8 g • Sugar: 22.8 g Sodium: 76.9 mg (without salt)

Ingredients:

- 2 medium ripe bananas, (the riper the better) sliced into 1/2" pieces 1 1/2 cup blueberries

- 1/4 cup honey

- 1 cup uncooked quick oats

- 1/4 cup chopped walnuts or pecans 1/2 tsp baking powder

- 3/4 tsp cinnamon 1 cup fat free milk 1 egg

- 1 tsp vanilla extract

Directions:

Preheat the oven to 375° F. Grease an 8x8 glass pan. Place the banana slices on the bottom of the dish in a single layer. Place half the blueberries on top of the bananas. Sprinkle with ¼ tsp of cinnamon, 1 T of honey and cover. Bake 15 min.

Combine the oats, half the nuts, and the remaining dry ingredients in a bowl. In a separate bowl, mix the milk, egg, honey and vanilla. Whisk till frothy.

Remove the bananas from the oven, pour the oats over the fruit for the second layer. Pour the wet mix over the oats, spreading evenly. Sprinkle the rest of the fruit and walnuts on top.

Bake for 30 minutes and serve warm.

Bountiful Banana Bread Oatmeal

303 calories, 9g total fat (1g sat fat), 268mg sodium, 45g carbs, 6.5g fiber, 10.5g sugars, 13.5g protein -- Smart Points : 7

Ingredients:

- 1/2 cup unsweetened vanilla almond milk 1/4 cup fat-free plain Greek yogurt

- 1 packet no-calorie sweetener (like Truvia) 1/8 tsp. cinnamon

- 1/8 tsp. vanilla extract 1/8 tsp. maple extract Dash salt

- 1/2 cup old-fashioned oats

- 1/4 cup mashed extra-ripe banana

- 1/4 oz. (about 1 tbsp.) chopped walnuts 2 T sugar-free syrup (optional)

Directions:

In a medium bowl, whisk the almond milk, yogurt, sweetener, cinnamon, vanilla extract, maple extract, and salt. Whisk until smooth. Stir in the oats and banana, making sure to saturate the oats with the liquid. Cover and refrigerate for 8 hours. Microwave before serving, then top with a drizzle of sugar free syrup and the walnuts. MAKES 1 SERVING

Breakfast Omelette in the Crock Pot

1/6th of recipe: 203 calories, 5.5g total fat (3g sat fat), 597mg sodium, 15g carbs, 3g fiber, 3g sugars, 21.5g protein -- Smart Points : 4

Ingredients:

- 4 cups roughly chopped cauliflower
- 3 frozen meatless or turkey sausage patties with 80 calories or less 2 cups frozen shredded hash browns
- 1 cup shredded reduced-fat Mexican blend cheese 3/4 cup chopped onion
- 3/4 cup chopped bell pepper
- 2 1/2 cups egg whites or fat-free liquid egg substitute 1/3 cup unsweetened plain almond milk
- 1/2 tsp. garlic powder
- 1/4 tsp. each salt and black pepper Optional toppings: salsa, light sour cream

Directions:

Blend cauliflower into rice-sized pieces, working in batches as needed.

Cook sausage patties per package directions, then crumble to bite sized pieces.

Fully line a slow cooker with heavy-duty aluminum foil, draping foil over the sides for a handle in the morning. Be sure to spray with nonstick spray.

Layer as follows, hash browns, sausage, ¾ cup cheese, cauliflower, onion and bell pepper. Whisk the eggs, milk and seasoning and pour over the mix in the crock pot. Cook on low for 8 hours.

Remove the lid, sprinkle the ¼ remaining cup of cheese. Cover and let sit while you get out the plates. Using the excess overlapping foil, lift the casserole out of the crock pot and serve with salsa and sour cream. Makes six servings.

Fruit and Fiber Smoothie

Calories: 180 • Servings: 2 • Size: 1-3/4 cup • Points +: 5 pts • Smart Points: 5

Ingredients:

- 1/2 cup raw quick oats 2 cups water

- 1/2 cup vanilla unsweetened almond milk 1/2 cup blueberries

- 1/2 ripe medium banana 1/2 tsp vanilla extract

- 2 tbsp raw sugar 1/2 cup ice

Directions:

In a blender combine all ingredients and blend until smooth. Makes 3 1/2 cups. 2 servings.

Gratifying Green Smoothie That is not Icky

1 serving

166 calories, 0.7 g fat, 0.0 g saturated fat, 37.5 g carbohydrates, 17.2 g sugar, 3.6 g protein, 7.5 g fiber, 37 mg sodium, 7 SmartPoints

Ingredients

- 1 cup frozen mixed berries
- 1 cup kale 1/2 banana 1 cup water

Directions:

Tear the kale into small pieces, removing them stems. Discard the stems. Put everything into the blender and pulse until smooth. For a thicker shake, use ice cubes instead of water.

Kale and Blueberry Smoothie

Servings: 1 • Size: 1 smoothie • Smart Points: 5

Calories: 312 • Fat: 12 g • Carb: 51 g • Fiber: 10 g • Protein: 9 g • Sugar: 31 g Sodium: 241 mg • Cholest: 0 mg

Ingredients:

- 3/4 cup organic frozen blueberries 1 loose cup baby kale

- 1 tbsp peanut butter (or any nut butter) 3/4 cup Unsweetened Vanilla Almond Milk 1/2 frozen ripe banana

- 2 pitted dates 1/2 cup ice

Directions:

Place all the ingredients into the blender and blend until smooth.

Piña Colada Smoothie with Banana

Servings: 1 • Smart Points: 4, Calories: 160 • Fat: 6 g • Carb: 27 g • Fiber: 4 g • Protein: 2g • Sugar: 18 g, Sodium: 95 mg • Cholesterol: 0 mg

Ingredients:

- 1/2 medium ripe frozen banana

- 6 oz Almond Breeze almond coconut milk

- 3 1/2 oz (about 1/2 cup) fresh pineapple 2/3 cup ice

- 1 T coconut flavoring

Directions: Place all the ingredients in the blender and blend until smooth.

Waffle and Ham Sandwiches

Calories 346, 4 total servings, Smart Points : 9

Ingredients

- 1/4 cup honey

- 2 Tbs butter or margarine

- 2 crisp, red apples, cored and sliced

- 8 frozen waffles, toasted

- 8 thin slices ham

Directions

Melt butter with 1/4 cup honey in a non-stick skillet, add apples and cook until they are done, about 6 minutes.

Toast waffles, top with ham and ¼ of the apples. Drizzle with sugar free maple syrup, if desired.

Serving Size is 2 waffles with toppings.

CHAPTER 5: SOUP AND SALAD RECIPES

Yummy soup and salad recipes that go great alongside your meals at lunch!

Beef and Barley Soup

Servings: 5 • Serving Size: 1 1/2 cups • Smart Points: 8

Calories: 336 • Fat: 11 g • Carbs: 27 g • Fiber: 6 g • Protein: 32 g • Sugar: 1.5 g Sodium: 453 mg

Ingredients:

- 1 tsp oil

- 1-1/2 lbs lean beef round stew meat

- 1 cup chopped carrots

- 1 cup chopped onions 1/2 cup chopped celery 2 cloves garlic, chopped 6 cups water

- 1 - 2 tsp kosher salt, to taste

- 2 bay leaves

- 2/3 cup dry barley

- fresh ground black pepper

Directions:

Brown meat in a large dutch oven with the oil. After the meat has browned, add carrots, onion, celery and garlic. Stir. Add the remaining ingredients except the barley and bring to a rolling boil. Reduce heat and simmer covered for 2 hours.

When meat is browned, add carrots, onion, celery and garlic to the pot and give it a good stir.

Add the barley, salt and pepper. Simmer until the barley is cooked, about 30 minutes, remove the bay leaves. Serve.

Beefy Tomato Italian Soup

Servings: 6 • Size: 1 generous cup • Smart Points: 5

Calories: 249 • Fat: 8 g • Carb: 23 g • Fiber: 3 g • Protein: 21 g
Sugar: 4 g • Sodium: 593 mg • Cholesterol: 49 mg

Ingredients:

- 1 lb 90% lean ground beef
- 1/2 teaspoon kosher salt 1/2 cup diced onion
- 1/2 cup diced celery 1/2 cup diced carrot
- 28 oz can diced tomatoes
- 32 oz beef stock

- 2 bay leaves
- 4 oz small pasta such as Acini di pepei grated parmesan cheese, optional

Directions:

In a Dutch oven, Brown the beef with the salt. Add the onions, celery and carrots and saute until the onions are translucent. Add the tomatoes, broth or stock and bay leaf, cover and cook low about 1 to 1 1/2 hours. Add the pasta, stir and cook 15 more minutes.

Buffalo (Hot Wing) Soup

yield: 11 (1 CUP) SERVINGS , SMARTPOINTS = 6 per (1 cup) serving

213 calories, 16 g carbs, 4 g sugars, 9 g fat, 5 g saturated fat, 17 g protein, 1 g fiber

Ingredients:

- 2 cups water
- 4 cups reduced sodium fat free chicken broth
- 1 lb uncooked boneless skinless chicken breasts

- 12 oz Russet potatoes, cubed

- 1 cup sliced carrots

- 1 cup chopped celery

- 1 cup flour

- teaspoon black pepper

- teaspoon salt

- 8 tablespoons (1 stick) of light butter

- 2 cups fat free half and half

- 4 oz 50% reduced fat sharp cheddar cheese, shredded

- 2 oz crumbled blue cheese

- 1/3 cup Buffalo wing sauce, or more to taste/drizzle on top

Directions:

Bring the water and chicken broth to a boil in a large Dutch oven. Add the chicken, potatoes, carrots and celery and simmer. Cover the pot and simmer for 25-30 minutes until chicken is done. Shred the chicken on a plate while the soup simmers.

Make a roux with the flour, salt and pepper. To make a roux: melt the butter over medium heat so as not to burn it. Stir in the flour mix a spoon at a time, mixing constantly. It will burn if it is not stirred constantly. Pour the half and half into the roux, stirring and stirring. Mixture will begin to thicken. Add the cheddar and blue cheeses and continue to cook, stirring while the cheeses are melted. Add in the wing sauce and stir to combine. Add the shredded chicken. Simmer for 10 minutes to thicken.

Cheeseburger Soup

yield: 5 (1 CUP + CROUTONS) SERVINGS, Smart Points: 8 per serving

259 calories, 16 g carbs, 5 g sugars, 10 g fat, 3 g saturated fat, 25 g protein, 1 g fiber

Ingredients:

- 1 ½ tablespoons light butter, divided
- 1 hamburger bun with sesame seeds A pinch of garlic powder and salt
- 1 celery stalk, diced
- 1 small onion, diced
- 2 garlic cloves, minced
- ¾ lb of 95% lean ground beef

- 1 ½ – 2 teaspoons McCormick Hamburger Seasoning

- 1 ½ cups fat free, low sodium beef broth

- 1 (10.75 oz) can of Campbell's Healthy Request Cheddar Cheese Soup

- 1 cup fat free plain Greek yogurt

- 3/4 cup shredded 2% sharp cheddar cheese, divided

Directions:

Pre-heat the oven to 325 degrees. Cut the hamburger bun into bite sized cubes, about 2 dozen. Melt 1 T of butter and toss the cubes in it to coat. Sprinkle with a dash of garlic powder and salt. Layer the cubes in a single layer on a baking sheet for 15 mins until crunchy. Set aside.

In a large pot, heat the remaining butter, add the celery and onion, cook until onion is translucent, add the garlic cook 4 more minutes. Remove the vegetables but save them. In the same pot, brown the ground beef, breaking it up as you cook, sprinkle with the seasoning and cook until brown.

Add the vegetables to the pot along with the broth, cheese soup, half and half, yogurt, and about 1/2 cup of the shredded cheese. Stir the mixture together and heat until the mixture starts to bubble, reduce the heat. Let simmer for 20 minutes. Serve topped with remaining cheese and croutons.

Clucky Quinoa Soup with Kale

Calories 284, per 1 ½ cup serving, 7 Smart points each serving

Ingredients

- 2 lbs boneless skinless chicken thighs

- 1 cup dry quinoa

- 4 cups kale, chopped

- 3 ribs celery, chopped

- 3 carrots, chopped

- 2 poblano peppers

- 1 onion, chopped finely

- 6 garlic cloves, minced

- 8 cup low sodium chicken broth 1/2 tsp cumin

- 1/2 tsp dried thyme Salt and pepper

Directions:

Cook in slow cooker on LOW for 8 hours.

Coconut Lime Thai Soup

6 servings Serving size is 1 1/2 cups Each serving = 3 Smart Points PER SERVING: 125 calories; 4g fat; 9g carbohydrates; 12g protein; 1.5g fiber

Ingredients

- 1 15 oz can light coconut milk
- 8 oz skinless, boneless chicken breast
- 2 cloves garlic, minced
- 2 tbsp fresh ginger, grated
- 1 small onion, halved and thinly sliced
- 1 head of bok choy, chopped
- 3 small pieces (about 3-5 inches long) of lemongrass stalks 5 cups fat free chicken broth
- 2 serrano peppers, diced
- 2 tsp sugar
- 1/3 cup fresh cilantro, chopped 3 tbsp fish sauce
- Juice from 4 limes

Directions:

Place a dutch oven over medium heat. Spray with cooking spray. Smash the lemongrass to release flavor. Add the onion, garlic, ginger, peppers and lemongrass to the dutch oven, along with ¼ cup of chicken broth. Cook 5 minutes until onions soften.

Stir in the chicken and broth. Boil, then reduce heat, cover and let simmer until chicken is done, approximately 10 minutes. Remove the chicken and shred, then return to the pot.

Stir in the lime juice, bok choy, fish sauce, sugar, coconut milk and cilantro. Cook for five minutes to tenderize the bok choy and blend the flavors. Remove the lemongrass and serve.

Split Pea Soup with Ham

Servings: 6 • Size: 1 1/4 cups • Smart Points: 8

Calories: 254 • Fat: 2 g • Carb: 51.5 g • Fiber: 20 g • Protein: 24 g • Sugar: 5 g Sodium: 694.5 mg

Ingredients:

- 1 lb dry green split peas

- 1 tsp olive oil

- 2 large carrots, peeled

- 1 medium onion, diced

- 2 cloves garlic, minced

- 7 oz reduced sodium ham steak, diced

- 8 cups water

- 1 tbsp Better Than Bouillon or 1 cube

- 1 bay leaf

Directions:

Rinse peas under cold water.

In a Dutch Oven, heat oil, add carrots, onions and garlic. Saute 5 minutes. Add remaining ingredients, simmer covered until peas are done, approximately 2 hours. Remove the bay leaf before serving.

Serve with crusty bread and a dollop of sour cream.

Salads:

Asian Chopped Salad with Sesame Dressing (In a Jar)

Servings: 4 • Size: 1 jar: 3 cups salad, 2 tbsp dressing • Smart Points: 7 , Calories: 231 • Fat: 13.5 g • Carb: 23 g • Fiber: 7.5 g • Protein: 8 g Sugar: 12 g • Sodium: 404 mg • Cholesterol: 0 mg

These will stay fresh in the refrigerator for a week.

Ingredients:

For Salad:

- 1 ½ cups shelled edamame or water chestnuts, sliced thinly

- 1 medium red bell pepper, thinly sliced then cut into 1-inch pieces

- 1 medium yellow bell pepper, thinly sliced then cut into 1-inch pieces 1 cup thinly sliced snow peas

- 1 cup shredded carrots

- 4 scallions, chopped

- 4 cups shredded purple cabbage (about 1/2 small head)

- 4 cups chopped Romaine lettuce (about 1 small head)

For Sesame Dressing:

- 2 tablespoons soy sauce

- 2 tablespoons lemon juice

- 2 teaspoons honey

- 1 teaspoon grated ginger

- 1 garlic clove, crushed

- 2 1/2 tablespoons oil

- 1/2 tablespoon sesame oil 1 teaspoon sesame seeds

Directions:

In a small mason jar combine the dressing ingredients and shake well.

Place 2 tablespoons of the dressing on the bottom of 4 large quart sized mason jars. Divide the water chestnuts or edamame and place over the dressing.

Then the peppers, carrots, snow peas, scallions, cabbage and lettuce and cover. Refrigerate until ready to eat. Shake well to toss then pour onto a plate.

Greek Cucumber Salad with Lemon and Feta

Servings: 1 • 1 salad • Smart Points: 7

Calories: 225 • Fat: 16 g • Carb: 16 g • Fiber: 4 g • Protein: 7 g • Sugar: 1 g Sodium: 697.5 mg • Cholesterol: 25 mg

Ingredients:

- 1/2 seedless English cucumber 1/4 of a green bell pepper, chopped 1/3 cup grape tomatoes, halved

- 5 pitted kalamata olives

- 1 tbsp red onion, sliced 1/2 fresh lemon

- 1 oz fresh feta, sliced thick

- 1/2 tablespoon extra virgin olive oil

- kosher salt and freshly ground black pepper 1/2 teaspoon fresh oregano leaves, minced

Directions: Dice the cucumbers into small cubes. Add the bell pepper, tomatoes, olives and red onion. In a small bowl, juice the lemon, add the olive oil, oregano, salt and pepper. Whisk the dressing and pour over the salad. Top with fresh feta.

Panzanella (Italian Bread Salad)

As a side dish: Servings: 8 • Serving Size: 1 cup • Smart Points: 3 pts Calories: 104.3 • Fat: 2.9 g • Protein: 3.1 g • Carb: 17.7 g • Fiber:2.2 g

As a main dish: Servings: 4 • Serving Size: 2 cups • Points: 6 pts

Ingredients:

- 8-10 medium ripe tomatoes, cut into 1 inch cubes 1 cup seedless cucumber, diced

- 1/2 red onion, chopped 8-10 basil leaves, chopped 1 tbsp extra virgin olive oil extra virgin olive oil spray

- 6 oz French bread or a good crusty Italian bread, sliced kosher salt and fresh ground pepper to taste

Directions:

Baste bread with olive oil and toast until nicely browned. Cut into 1 inch cubes. Set aside.

In a large bowl, combine the tomatoes, cucumber, red onion, basil, olive oil, salt and pepper. Let it rest for 30 minutes to let the flavors meld. Add the bread cubes and toss together.

Pear Salad with Fresh Greens

Serving size is about 1 2/3 cups, Each serving = 4 Smart Points

149 calories; 9.7g fat; 2.6g saturated fat; 15g carbohydrates; 7g sugar; 3.4g protein; 3.6g fiber

Ingredients

- 6 cups mixed baby lettuce & spinach leaves

- 2 medium pears sliced

- 1/4 cup blue cheese crumbled or chopped 4 Tbsp balsamic vinegar

- 4 tsp maple syrup salt to taste

- 2 Tbsp olive oil

- 1 Tbsp pine nuts optional

Directions:

Combine the vinegar, syrup, salt and olive oil. Mix well.

Combine the lettuce and pears. Drizzle the dressing and the blue cheese onto the salad components. Toss and sprinkle with pine nuts.

Shrimp and Watermelon Salad

Servings: 4 • Size: 1 salad • Smart Points: 7

Calories: 293 • Fat: 18 g • Carb: 12 g • Fiber: 2 g • Protein: 22 g • Sugar: 7 g Sodium: 257 mg • Cholesterol: 121 mg

Ingredients: For the dressing:

- 2 1/2 tbsp DeLallo golden balsamic vinegar

- 1 tsp water

- 1 tbsp chopped shallots 1/8th tsp kosher salt pinch fresh black pepper 2 tbsp extra virgin olive oil

For the shrimp:

- 10 oz shelled and deveined (about 24) large shrimp

- 1 clove garlic crushed seasoned salt, to taste

For the Salad:

- 8 cups chopped romaine

- 4 cups diced watermelon

- 4 ounces soft goat cheese

Directions:

In a bowl, whisk vinegar, water, shallots, salt and pepper. Add olive oil, stirring until smooth.

For the shrimp:

Season shrimp with seasoned salt, then mix in crushed garlic.

Prepare the skillet with oil, when hot grill or saute the shrimp about 1 to 2 minutes on each side. Set aside.

Toss the romaine with the dressing. Divide on four plates, layer with watermelon, goat cheese and grilled shrimp.

Tomato Salad

Servings: 4 • Smart Points: 2 , Calories: 110.6 • Fat: 9.1 g • Carb: 7.6 g • Fiber: 1.5 g • Protein: 1.2 g • Sugar: 0 g Sodium: 139.1 mg

Ingredients:

- 4 medium ripe tomatoes, sliced 1/4 cup red onion, chopped

- 2 tbsp extra virgin olive oil

- 8 kalamata olives fresh basil, sliced

- kosher salt and fresh pepper

Directions:

In a bowl combine onions, olive oil, salt and pepper. Marinate about 5-10 minutes. Slice the tomatoes and arrange in a pleasing manner on a serving plate. Pour olive oil and onions on top and salt and pepper. Top with fresh basil. Divide equally in 4 plates.

Chapter 6: Appetizers and Main Dishes

Delicious appetizers and main course meals that are simple to make!

Appetizers:

BLT Dip

yield: 16 (1/3 CUP) servings, Smart Points: 5 per (1/3 cup) serving

134 calories, 2 g carbs, 1 g sugars, 9 g fat, 6 g saturated fat, 8 g protein, 0 g fiber

Ingredients:

- 12 slices center cut bacon
- 2 (8 oz) blocks of 1/3 less fat cream cheese 2/3 cup fat free sour cream
- 4 oz 50% reduced fat sharp cheddar cheese, shredded (about 1 cup) 5 oz (1 ¼ cups) shredded 2% Mozzarella cheese
- 1 tablespoon yellow mustard

- teaspoon Italian seasoning

- teaspoon garlic powder Salt & pepper to taste

- 1 cup diced, seeded tomatoes

- 1 ½ cups shredded iceberg lettuce

Directions:

Cook the bacon until crisp and crumble into small pieces. Set aside on paper towels. Pre-heat the oven to 350. Lightly grease or spray an 8x8 dish. Combine the cream cheese, sour cream, cheddar, Mozzarella, mustard, Italian seasoning, garlic powder, ¼ cup of the crumbled bacon, salt and

pepper and mix with a mixer. Place the mixture into the bottom of the 8x8 dish. Spread evenly. Bake for 25-30 minutes.

Take it out of the oven and top with the remaining bacon crumbles, the diced tomatoes and the shredded lettuce. Serve hot.

Buffalo Wing Hummus

yield: 8 (1/4 CUP) SERVINGS, Smart Points: 2 per serving

72 calories, 12 g carbs, 1 g sugars, 2 g fat, 0 g saturated fat, 3 g protein, 2 g fiber

Ingredients:

- 1 ½ cups canned chickpeas, drained and rinsed (reserve ¼ cup of the liquid from the can)

- 2 cloves garlic

- 2 tablespoons tahini

- 2 tablespoons fresh lemon juice ¾ teaspoon paprika

- 1 tablespoon barbecue sauce

- 1 ½ tablespoons Frank's Red Hot (or similar cayenne pepper sauce)

- 1 ½ teaspoons white vinegar ¾ teaspoon salt

Directions:

Combine all ingredients including the reserved liquid into a blender. Blend until smooth. Serve.

Chicken Philly Cheesesteak Dip

Servings: 12 • Size: scant 1/4 cup • Smart Points: 3

Calories: 125 • Fat: 9 g • Saturated Fat: 4 g • Carb: 3 g • Fiber: 0 g • Protein: 8 g Sugar: 1 g • Sodium: 234 mg • Cholesterol: 28 mg

Ingredients:

- 8 ounces thin sliced chicken cutlets 1/8 teaspoon kosher salt

- black pepper to taste cooking spray

- 1 cup diced onion

- 1 cup diced green pepper 1/4 cup light mayonnaise 1/2 cup light sour cream

- 4 oz light cream cheese, softened

- 4 oz shredded mild provolone cheese

Directions:

Season chicken with salt and pepper. Cook on high heat until cooked through. Slice thinly.

Saute onions and peppers in oil for 5-10 minutes, until onions are translucent. Preheat oven to 350°F.

Combine all the ingredients in an oven-proof dish and bake 20-25 minutes, until cheese is melted.

Hot & Cheesy Bean Dip

yield: 12 (1/3 CUP) Servings, Smart Points: 4 per (1/3 cup) serving

106 calories, 8 g carbs, 2 g sugars, 6 g fat, 4 g saturated fat, 6 g protein, 2 g fiber

Ingredients:

- 8 oz of 1/3 less fat cream cheese, softened ½ cup fat free sour cream
- 16 oz can of fat free refried beans
- 1 tablespoon green chilies
- teaspoon chili powder 1 teaspoon cumin
- ¼ teaspoon salt
- cup salsa
- 4 oz of reduced fat sharp cheddar cheese, shredded

Directions:

Preheat the oven to 350. Combine the cream cheese, softened, and the sour cream. Mix until smooth and place in the bottom of a glass pie plate. Combine the beans and spices, spread over the cream cheese mix. Spread the salsa over this layer, top with cheese.

Bake for 30 minutes and serve.

Light Brie & Jam

yield: 4 Servings, Smart Points: 4 per serving

Ingredients:

- 7 oz President Light Brie

- 1/3 cup Smucker's Sugar Free Jam (I used Blackberry)

Directions:

Remove the rind off the top surface of the cheese with a sharp knife. Spread 1/3 c of jam onto surface of the brie. Microwave for about 1 minute or until warmed through. Serve with toasted points of very thinly sliced bread.

Loaded Potato Rounds

yield: 6, Smart Points: 5 per (1/6th) serving Nutritional Information: 167 calories, 20 g carbs, 1 g sugars, 7 g fat, 3 g saturated fat, 6 g protein, 3 g fiber

Ingredients:

- 3 slices uncooked center cut bacon, diced

- 1 ½ lbs Russet Potatoes, scrubbed (for me this was about 2 large potatoes) 5 teaspoons olive oil

- sea salt, to taste

- 2/3 cup 2% shredded cheddar 1-2 scallions, sliced (greens only)

Directions:

Preheat the oven to 425 degrees.

Cook the bacon quickly until bacon pieces are crisp. Remove the bacon pieces to a paper towel stack using a slotted spoon and set aside.

Cut the potatoes into 1/4" thick slices. Drizzle with olive oil and sprinkle with salt. Bake for 35-40 minutes until potatoes are golden.

Remove the potatoes from the oven, top with the shredded cheese and bacon. Broil for 2 minutes until the cheese is melted. Sprinkle with green onions and serve.

Mushroom Flatbreads with a Trio of Cheese

yield: 1 Flatbread , Smart Points: 8 per flatbread

265 calories, 12 g carbs, 3 g sugars, 11 g fat, 4 g saturated fat, 24 g protein, 9 g fiber

Ingredients:

- 1 ½ oz sliced mushrooms (I used Baby Bellas)
- teaspoon dried parsley flakes 1/8 teaspoon dried marjoram
- teaspoon minced garlic
- 1 Flatout Light Original Flatbread
- 2 wedges of The Laughing Cow Creamy Swiss Garlic & Herb cheese, softened to room temperature
- oz 2% shredded Mozzarella cheese
- oz Parmesan cheese, finely shredded Freshly cracked black pepper, to taste

Directions:

Pre-heat the oven to 350. Spray a skillet and toast the mushrooms, parsley and marjoram together until browned. Add the garlic and cook for 30 seconds. Set aside. Bake the flatbread directly on the middle rack for 3 ½ min, until firm. Remove from the oven, spread with the soft cheese, sprinkle with mozzarella, top with the seasoned mushroom mix. Sprinkle with the parmesan and black pepper to suit. Bake in the middle rack for 5 minutes until the edges are brown. Slice and serve.

Pepperoni Bites

yield: 6 (4 BITE) SERVINGS, Smart Points 6 per serving of 4 bites

210 calories, 23 g carbs, 3 g sugar, 9 g fat, 3 g saturated fat, 11 g protein, 1 g fiber

Ingredients:

- 10 oz can refrigerated pizza crust dough

- 1 cup shredded reduced fat mozzarella cheese

- 2 oz sliced turkey pepperoni

- 1 tablespoon Extra Virgin Olive Oil

- 1 tablespoon Grated Parmesan Cheese Italian Seasonings to taste

Directions:

Pre-heat the oven to 400. Spray a glass pie plate. Unroll pizza crust and cut into 24 pieces. Flatten it and place 2 tsp of cheese in the center, place a piece of pepperoni (reg size, more if the tiny ones) on top of the cheese, fold into a ball. Place the ball, seam side down, on the pie plate. Continue with 23 more. Brush the olive oil on top of the bites, sprinkle with Parm and Italian seasoning. Bake for 20 minutes until done.

Spinach and Artichoke Dip

Servings: 15 • Serving Size: 1/4 cup • Smart Points: 2 , Calories: 73 • Fat: 4.5 g • Carb: 3.5 g • Fiber: 1 g • Protein: 5 g • Sugar: 0.6 g Sodium: 245 g

Ingredients:

- 13.75 oz artichoke hearts packed in water, drained

- 10 oz frozen spinach, thawed and squeezed 1/4 cup chopped shallots

- 1 clove garlic

- 1/2 cup fat free Greek yogurt 1/2 cup light mayonnaise 2/3 cup Parmigiano Reggiano

- 4 oz shredded part skim mozzarella cheese salt and fresh pepper to taste

- olive oil spray

Directions:

Preheat oven to 375°F.

Coarsely chop the artichoke hearts, garlic and shallots.

Place in an oven-proof dish and bake at 375° for 20-25 minutes, until cheese is melted. Serve right away.

Makes about 3-3/4 cups.

Zucchini Fries with Marinara Sauce

yield: 3 SERVINGS, Smart Points: 4 per serving with sauce, 3 without sauce

Ingredients:

Baked Zucchini Fries:

- 3 medium zucchini sliced into 3″ x 1/2″ sticks

- 1 large egg white

- 1/3 cup seasoned bread crumbs

- 2 tablespoons grated Pecorino Romano cheese 1/4 teaspoons garlic powder

- salt

- black pepper cooking spray

Marinara Sauce:

- 1 tsp olive oil

- 2 cloves garlic, minced

- 1 (28 oz) can crushed tomatoes

- 1 small bay leaf

- 1 teaspoon oregano

- 2 Tablespoon chopped fresh basil salt and black pepper to taste

Directions:

Preheat oven to 425. Heat a pan with the olive oil and saute garlic until golden. Add the tomatoes and the rest of the marinara sauce ingredients. Stir until well mixed, then simmer covered for 20 minutes.

Beat the egg in a bowl, sprinkle with salt and pepper. Combine breadcrumbs, garlic powder and cheese in a shallow bowl. (I use a pie plate.)

Spray a baking sheet sheet with cooking spray and set to the side.

Dip zucchini sticks into eggs and then into the bread crumb and cheese mixture to coat. Place the zucchini fries on the baking sheet in a single layer, spray with more cooking, then bake at 425F for 25 minutes. Serve with marinara sauce.

Main Dishes

Baked Chicken Parmesan

Servings: 8 • Serving Size: 1 piece • Smart Points 5

Calories: 251 • Fat: 9.5 g • Protein: 31.5 g • Carb: 14 g • Fiber: 1.5 g • Sugar: 0 Cholesterol: 14 mg

Ingredients:

- 4 (about 8 oz each) chicken breast, fat trimmed, sliced in half to make 8 3/4 cup seasoned breadcrumbs

- 1/4 cup grated Parmesan cheese 2 tbsp butter, melted (or olive oil)

- 3/4 cup reduced fat mozzarella cheese (I used Polly-o) 1 cup marinara

- cooking spray

Directions:

Preheat oven to 450°. Spray a large cooking sheet with spray.

Combine breadcrumbs and parmesan cheese in a pie plate. Melt the butter and brush the butter onto the chicken, then coat with the crumb mixture. Place on baking sheet in a single layer. Repeat until all the chicken is on the sheet. Drizzle with oil and bake 20 minutes. Turn the chicken and bake another 5 minutes.

Remove from oven, top with 1 tbsp sauce over each piece of chicken and 1 1/2 tbsp of shredded mozzarella cheese.

Bake until cheese is melted.

Bacon BBQ Cheeseburger Quesadillas

yield: 5 QUESADILLAS, SMARTPOINTS: 8 per quesadilla

297 calories, 20 g carbs, 4 g sugars, 11 g fat, 5 g saturated fat, 31 g protein, 3 g fiber

Ingredients:

- ½ cup chopped onion

- 1 lb 95% lean ground beef

- 1 tablespoon McCormick Hamburger seasoning

- 4 tablespoons barbecue sauce

- 3 strips crispy cooked center cut bacon, chopped

- 10 small corn tortillas (I use Mission Extra Thin Yellow Corn Tortillas) 5 oz 50% reduced fat sharp cheddar cheese, shredded

Directions:

Place chopped onions into a sprayed skillet and cook until translucent. Add the ground beef until meat is cooked thoroughly and broken into small bite-sized pieces. Drain. Add the hamburger seasoning, barbecue sauce and bacon, stir until well combined. Remove from heat.

Spray one side of five tortillas and place sprayed side down in a skillet or griddle. Sprinkle 1 T shredded cheese onto the surface of each tortilla and top with ½ cup of the

meat mixture. Spread the meet out on the tortilla, then cover with another tablespoon of cheese. Spray one side of 5 more tortillas and stack onto the meat with the spray side up. Turn the heat up on the pan and toast on one side until the cheese is melted, then flip to the other side. Cut into quarters and serve hot with extra salsa.

Black Pepper Chicken

Yields: 6 servings | Serving Size: 1 cup | Calories: 199 | Total Fat: 8 g | Saturated Fat: 1 g | Trans Fat: 0 g | Cholesterol: 83 mg | Sodium: 341 mg | Carbohydrates: 4 g | Dietary Fiber: 1 g | Sugars: 2 g | Protein: 27 g | SmartPoints: 4 |

Ingredients

- 1-1/2 pounds boneless, skinless chicken breasts, cut into cubes 1 red bell pepper, seeded and cut into strips

- 1-1/2 teaspoons freshly ground black pepper 1-inch fresh ginger root, peeled and finely chopped 2 cloves garlic, peeled and finely minced

- 3 tablespoons lite soy sauce, divided

- 3 tablespoons white vinegar, divided

- 1 tablespoon honey

- 2 tablespoons olive oil

Directions

Whisk together half of the soy sauce, vinegar, and sweetener. Add the chicken and toss to coat. Marinate for 30 minutes in the fridge.

Add oil to a skillet and the garlic and ginger. Cook for 30 seconds, just until garlic is golden.

Add the marinated chicken with the marinade and cook for 3 minutes. Add the remaining ingredients and cook about 10 minutes. Make sure the chicken is done. Serve.

Cajun Red Beans and Rice

Yields: 6 servings | Calories: 307 | Total Fat: 7g | Saturated Fat: 2g | Trans Fat: 0g | Cholesterol: 33mg | Sodium: 721mg | Carbohydrates: 43g | Fiber: 6g | Sugar: 4g | Protein: 17g | SmartPoints: 9 |

Ingredients

- 1 pound lean turkey sausage

- 1 cup (uncooked) 10-minute brown rice

- 1 tablespoon extra-virgin olive oil

- 1 clove garlic, crushed

- 1 medium onion, coarsely chopped

- 1 medium red bell pepper, coarsely chopped

- 2 (15-ounce) cans red beans

- 1 cup vegetable broth

- 2 bay leaves

- 1/4 teaspoon kosher or sea salt 1/8 teaspoon ground pepper

Directions

For rice and beans:

Cook brown rice per package directions. Leave covered until ready to serve.

In a large skillet, sauté sausages over medium heat until they are done. Add oil if necessary. Move sausages to one side of saucepan. Sauté onions, and bell pepper until tender, or about 4 minutes. Add garlic and sauté 1 additional minute.

Add red beans, vegetable broth, and bay leaves, give it a good stir. Cook for about 5 minutes. Sauce will thicken.

Serve over brown rice.

Cheesy Taco Pasta

10 SmartPoints per serving, 376 calories, 37 g carbs, 5 g sugars, 13 g fat, 6 g saturated fat, 29 g protein, 6 g fiber, yield: 6 (1 ROUNDED CUP) SERVINGS

Ingredients:

- 8 oz wheat pasta (I used Barilla medium shells)

- 1 lb 95% lean ground beef

- 1 oz packet reduced sodium taco seasoning

- 1 ½ cups chunky salsa ½ cup water

- ¼ cup fat free sour cream

- cup shredded 2 % reduced fat cheddar cheese

- cup shredded sharp cheddar cheese (I used extra sharp) Salt & pepper to taste

Directions:

Cook pasta per package instructions. Cook the ground beef, drain the beef, add the taco seasoning, salsa and water. Simmer until the sauce has thickened. Drain the pasta and mix in with the beef. Add the cheese and sour cream, salt and pepper. Serve with lettuce and tomato.

Chicken & Pasta Recipe

Yields: 6 servings | Serving Size: 1 1/2 cups | Calories: 337 | Total Fat: 13g | Saturated Fat: 4g | Trans Fat: 0g | Cholesterol:

37mg | Sodium: 432mg | Carbohydrates: 38g | Fiber: 6g | Sugar: 1g | Protein: 20g | Smart Points: 10 |

Ingredients

- 1/2 pound boneless, skinless chicken breast, chopped into bite-size(1-inch) pieces 3 tablespoons extra-virgin olive oil

- 1/2 teaspoon kosher or sea salt 3 cloves garlic, thinly sliced

- 1 cup sliced mushrooms

- 1 cup (1/2 pint) cherry or grape tomatoes, sliced in half 10 ounces whole wheat or high protein spaghetti

- 1/2 cup chopped fresh basil leaves 1/4 teaspoon black pepper

- 3/4 cup freshly grated Parmesan cheese

Directions

Cook chicken pieces and mushrooms in a large skillet in the olive oil, about 10 minutes. Add the garlic and tomatoes and cook a minute more.

Cook the spaghetti until al dente. Drain the pasta except ½ cup of water. Mix the pasta and the chicken with vegetables. Sprinkle with the olive oil and parmesan cheese.

Crock Pot Chicken Taco Chili

Servings: 10 • Serving Size: about 1 cup • Smart Points: 5

Calories: 209 • Fat: 3 g • Sat Fat: 0 g • Protein: 23 g • Carb: 26 g • Fiber: 7 g Sugar: 4 g • Sodium: 867 mg • Cholesterol: 50 mg

Ingredients:

- 1 small onion, chopped
- 1 (15.5 oz) can black beans
- 1 (15.5 oz) can kidney beans
- 1 (8 oz) can tomato sauce
- 10 oz package frozen corn kernels
- 2 (10 oz) cans diced tomatoes w/chilies
- 4 oz can chopped green chili peppers, chopped
- 1 packet reduced sodium taco seasoning
- 1 tbsp cumin
- 1 tbsp chili powder
- 24 oz (3-4) boneless skinless chicken breasts 1/4 cup chopped fresh cilantro

Directions:

Combine all ingredients in a crock pot. Make sure the chicken is covered with the liquid. Cook on LOW for 8 to 10 hours or on HIGH for 4 to 6 hours. Before serving, remove chicken and shred. Stir into the chili and serve.

Creamy Italian Chicken in Crockpot

Calories 374, ¾ cup serving, 12 Smart Points

Ingredients

- 4 chicken breasts
- 1 (8 oz) cream cheese, softened
- 1 can cream of chicken
- 1 dry packet of italian seasoning

Directions

Layer in Crockpot, cook on low for 4-6 hours

Eggplant Parmesan with Chicken

1/4th of pan (4" X 4"): 350 calories, 12g total fat (5.5g sat fat), 814mg sodium, 14.5g carbs, 6g fiber, 7.5g sugars, 45.5g protein -- Smart Points = 6

Ingredients:

- 1 large eggplant (about 20 oz.), ends removed

- Four 5-oz. boneless skinless chicken breast cutlets, pounded to 1/4-inch thickness 1 cup canned crushed tomatoes

- 1 cup shredded part-skim mozzarella cheese 1/4 cup grated Parmesan cheese

- Seasonings: garlic powder, onion powder, salt, Italian seasoning

Directions:

Preheat oven to 400 degrees. Spray 2 baking sheets and an 8" X 8" baking pan to grease. Slice the eggplant lengthwise into slices ½ inch thick. Sprinkle the eggplant with ½ tsp. garlic powder, ½ tsp onion powder and ¼ tsp salt, place in a single lay on one of the baking pans. Lay the chicken cutlets on the other baking pan and sprinkle with same spices, ½ tsp. garlic powder, ½ tsp onion powder and ¼ tsp salt. Bake the chicken and the eggplant for 20 minutes.

To make the sauce: Add tomatoes, 1 ½ tsp Italian seasoning and ½ tsp garlic powder and ½ tsp onion powder and mix well. This can be mixed in a bowl.

Take the chicken out of the oven. Flip the eggplant and cook it 12 more minutes. Leave the oven on.

In the 8x8 pan, layer the sauce, the eggplant, the sauce, mozzarella cheese, Parm cheese, sauce, chicken, eggplant, sauce, mozzarella cheese, Parm cheese. Cover and bake for 30 minutes. Remove the foil and brown the cheese. Cool 10 minutes before slicing to let the flavors meld.

Jerked Shrimp Tropical Skewers

Makes about 9 skewers

One skewer is 121 calories, 1.0 g fat, 0.0 g saturated fat, 14.5 g carbohydrates, 5.6 g sugar, 13.2 g protein, 0.8 g fiber, 139 mg sodium, 3 SmartPoints

Ingredients

- 1 pound small shrimp (25-30 count), peeled ½ cup jerk marinade (for example Lawry's)

- 1 fresh pineapple, peeled and cut into 1-inch chunks

Directions:

Peel the shrimp and place in the marinade for 30 minutes in the fridge. Alternate between the pineapple chunks and the shrimp as you place on skewers.

Grill the skewers on for about 2 minutes, then flip. Shrimp is bright pink when done.

Lemony Chicken and Asparagus Stir Fry

Servings: 4 • Size: 1 1/4 cups • Points +: 6 pts • Smart Points: 4

Calories: 268 • Fat: 7 g • Carb: 10 g • Fiber: 3 g • Protein: 41 g • Sugar: 0 g Sodium: 437 mg (without salt) • Cholest: 98 mg

Ingredients:

1 1/2 pounds skinless chicken breast, cut into 1-inch cubes Kosher salt, to taste

1/2 cup reduced-sodium chicken broth 2 tablespoons reduced-sodium soy sauce 2 teaspoons cornstarch

2 tablespoons water

1 tbsp oil, divided

1 bunch asparagus, ends trimmed, cut into 2-inch pieces 6 cloves garlic, chopped

1 tbsp fresh ginger

3 tablespoons fresh lemon juice fresh black pepper, to taste

Directions:

Lightly salt the chicken. In a small bowl, mix and stir the chicken broth and soy sauce. In a second small bowl combine the cornstarch and water, mix well to combine.

Heat a large non-stick wok or skillet, when hot add 1 teaspoon of the oil, and the asparagus and cook 3 to 4 minutes. Add the garlic and ginger, cook until the ginger is golden, about 1 minute. Set it to the side.

Turn heat to high, add 1 teaspoon of oil and half of the chicken. Cook until browned and cooked through, 4 minutes on each side. Repeat with the remaining oil and chicken. Set aside.

Add the soy sauce mixture; bring to a boil and cook about 1-1/2 minutes. Add lemon juice and cornstarch mixture, it will thicken slightly. Add the chicken and asparagus, mix well and serve.

Lime and Pork Cutlets

Servings: 4 • Size: 1 cutlet • Smart Points: 7

Calories: 216 • Fat: 10 g • Saturated Fat: 2 g • Carb: 11 g • Fiber: 1 g • Protein: 36 g Sugar: 1 g • Sodium: 404 mg • Cholesterol: 89 mg

Ingredients:

- 4 (5 oz) thin sliced lean pork sirloin cutlets seasoned salt

- 2 large egg whites, beaten 1/2 teaspoon sazon (Goya)

- 1/2 cup seasoned breadcrumbs 1 1/2 tbsp olive oil

- lime wedges for serving

Directions:

Season pork cutlets with 3/4 teaspoon seasoning salt. Place breadcrumbs in a shallow bowl. In a different bowl, beat egg whites with sazon. Dip cutlets in egg whites, then breadcrumb mixture.

Heat a frying pan, add the olive oil and pork cutlets, cook about 6 minutes on each side, until golden brown. Squeeze half a lime over the cutlets. Serve with remaining lime wedges.

Seasoned Chicken with Roasted Vegetables

Servings: 4 • Size: 2 thighs + vegetables • Smart Points: 8

Calories: 401 • Fat: 17 g • Saturated Fat: 3 g • Carb: 15 g • Fiber: 4 g • Protein: 48 g Sugar: 2 g • Sodium: 518 mg • Cholesterol: 214 mg

Ingredients:

- 8 (4 oz each) boneless skinless chicken thighs, trimmed of fat 1 teaspoon kosher salt

- fresh black pepper, to taste cooking spray

- 10 medium asparagus, ends trimmed, cut in half

- 2 red bell peppers

- 1 red onions, chopped in large chunks

- 1/2 cup carrots, sliced in half long, cut into 3-inch pieces 5 oz sliced mushrooms

- 1/4 cup plus 1 tbsp balsamic vinegar 2 tablespoons extra virgin olive oil

- 2 cloves garlic, smashed and roughly chopped 1/2 tsp sugar

- 1 1/2 tablespoons fresh rosemary 1/2 tbsp dried oregano or thyme 2 leaves fresh sage, chopped

Directions:

Preheat oven to 425°F. Season the chicken with salt and pepper. Spray 2 large baking sheets with oil.

Combine all the ingredients together in a large bowl, then coat chicken and vegetables with the mixture. Place on the baking sheets in a single layer. Do not allow anything to touch. Bake 25 minutes.

Slow Cooked Sesame Beef for Lettuce Wraps

Calories: 215, serving size ½ cup, 4 Smart Points

Ingredients

- 2 lb extra lean top round beef roast

- 2 tbsp soy sauce

- 2 tbsp sesame oil

- 2 tbsp rice wine vinegar

- 1 tbsp tomato paste (or ketchup)

- 1 tbsp brown sugar (or 1 packet Stevia)

- 2 tbsp fresh ginger, grated

- 4 garlic cloves, minced 1/2 cup onion, diced

- 1/4 cup sesame seeds, divided (regular, black, or a mix of both) 1/4 cup beef broth

Directions

Place the beef in the bottom of the crock pot. Whisk together the remaining ingredients and pour on top the beef. Cook on LOW for 6-8 hours. Remove beef and shred. Stir back into sauce and serve in lettuce cups, ¼ cup per lettuce leaf. 2 leaves equals one serving.

Slow Cooker Stuffed Cabbage Rolls

Yields: 6 servings | Serving Size: 2 cabbage rolls | Calories: 218 | Total Fat: 7 g | Saturated Fat: 2 g | Trans Fat: 0 g | Cholesterol: 93 mg | Sodium: 201 mg | Carbohydrates: 23 g | Dietary Fiber: 3 g | Sugars: 12 g | Protein: 17 g | Smart Points: 7 |

Ingredients For the rolls:

- 12 leaves cabbage

- 1 cup cooked long grain rice

- 1 egg, beaten 1/4 cup milk

- 1/4 cup finely chopped white or yellow onion 1 clove finely chopped garlic

- 1 pound raw, lean ground turkey

For the sauce:

- 1 1/4 teaspoons salt

- 1 1/4 teaspoons ground black pepper

- 1 (15-ounce) can tomato sauce

- 2 tablespoons ketchup

- 1 teaspoon Worcestershire sauce

- 1 teaspoon paprika

- 2 tablespoons lemon juice

- 2 tablespoons honey

- 1/2 teaspoon dried thyme leaves

Directions

Boil cabbage leaves for 2 minutes in hot salted water. Mix together tomato sauce, lemon juice, ketchup, honey, spices, Worcestershire sauce, and the salt and pepper.

In a separate bowl, place the cooked rice, ground turkey and egg, milk, onion, garlic. Add 1/4 of the tomato sauce and spices and mix well.

Scoop about 2 heaping tablespoons of the rice/turkey mix into the center of each cabbage roll. Roll up the leaves and tuck the ends like a burrito. Top with the tomato sauce mixture and cover.

Cook on low for 8 to 9 hours or on high for 4 to 5 hours.

Sticky and Sweet Chicken Thighs

Calories 241, serving size 2 thighs, 6 Smart Points

Ingredients

- ½ cup no sugar added grape jelly, apricot and plum is good also

- 1/2 cup ketchup

- 1/2 cup onions, diced 2 tbsp white vinegar 1 tsp dry mustard

- 2 lbs. boneless skinless chicken thighs (12 thighs)

Directions

Put everything in a sauce pan but the chicken and bring to a boil to thicken. Preheat oven to 400F.

Place chicken in a greased, glass baking dish. Pour sauce over to cover. Bake for 45 minutes.

CHAPTER 7: DELICIOUS DESSERTS

Just because you have goals to lose fat does not at all mean you should eliminate desserts from your diet. As long as you are in a CALORIE DEFICIT every day you will lose the weight you want and because of that you can include yummy desserts into your diet!

Berries & Cream Dessert Cups

yield: 12 CUPS, Smart Points: 3 per cup

87 calories, 14 g carbs, 8 g sugars, 2 g fat, 1 g saturated fat, 3 g protein, 1 g fiber

Ingredients:

- 12 wonton wrappers

- 5 teaspoons sugar

- 1 teaspoon cinnamon

- 4 oz 1/3 less fat cream cheese

- 1 cup vanilla nonfat Greek yogurt ½ teaspoon vanilla extract

- 4 tablespoons sugar

- 1 ¼ cup fresh berries

Directions:

Pre-heat the oven to 350. Lightly spray a muffin tin. Set aside. Mix together the 5 teaspoons of sugar and the cinnamon.

On a sheet of parchment paper, lay out the wonton wrappers. Lightly spray the wrappers and then sprinkle each with ¼ teaspoon of the cinnamon sugar. Flip each wrapper over repeating so that each side is covered. Push each wonton wrapper into a cup of the muffin tray to make a cup. Bake in the oven for 8 minutes, they will be brown.

Mix the cream cheese, yogurt, vanilla extract, and the remaining 4 tablespoons of sugar with a mixer until smooth. Place 1 heaping T of filling into each cinnamon cup, top with berries and serve immediately.

Blueberry Mango Frozen Treats

8 servings, Serving size is about 1/2 cup, 2 Smart Points, 86 calories

Ingredients

- 1 cup fresh or thawed blueberries

- 1 cup fresh or thawed mango chunks

- 1 1/2 cups plain Greek yogurt, non-fat

- 1 medium banana

- 2 – 3 Tbsp honey, or to taste

- 2 limes, juiced

- Popsicle molds, or paper cups and sticks

Directions

Place all the ingredients in a blender, with the addition of 1 cup of water. Blend until smooth. Divide into the molds or cups. Place the sticks and freeze for 4 hours.

Caramel Apple Crisp Fingers

Calories 77... Fat 1.2g... Saturated fat 0.1g... Carbs 15.2g...

Fiber 0.5g... Sugars 3.8g... Protein 1.8g, 3 Smart Points

Ingredients

- 1 pillsbury pizza dough

- 3 peeled and diced apples (your choice)

- 1 Tbsp white sugar ½ tsp cinnamon

- Topping
- 1 cup flour
- 1 cup oats
- 2 Tbsp brown sugar
- 1 tsp cinnamon
- 2 Tbsp light margarine, softened
- 2 Tbsp sugar free caramel sauce

Directions

Preheat oven to 350F, spray a cookie sheet and unroll your pizza dough, place on the sheet. Bake pizza dough 4 minutes, remove from oven, lower the oven temperature to 325F.

Mix the diced apples, white sugar, and ½ tsp cinnamon together. Spread over pizza dough.

Mix your oats, flour, brown sugar, 1 Tbsp cinnamon and margarine together, crumble over the apples.

Bake in oven for 18 minutes. Immediately after it comes out of oven drizzle with caramel topping. Use a pizza cutter and cut horizontally across the middle and then 10 cuts vertical to leave you with 20 pizza fingers.

Cheesecake Parfait

Makes 6 servings Nutrition Information Per Serving: Calories 185 : Fat 8 grams (Sat. 5 gm) : Carbohydrate 20 (Sugar 8 gm) : Fiber 2 grams : Protein 7 grams : Sodium 280 milligrams : Smart Points: 6 Points

Ingredients

- ½ cup graham-cracker crumbs (regular or chocolate)

- 2 tablespoons granulated no-calorie sweetener* or 3 packets 1 ½ tablespoons butter

- 4 ounces tub-style light cream cheese

- 4 ounces nonfat cream cheese, room temperature ½ cup light sour cream

- ¼ cup granulated no-calorie sweetener* or 6 packets 1 cup light whipped topping, thawed

- 1 1/2 cups thawed blueberries, strawberries, or thawed frozen dark cherries

Directions

Select 6 tall, stemmed glasses. Mix graham-cracker crumbs, 2 tablespoons sweetener, and butter. Set aside.

Beat cream cheeses with an electric mixer until smooth. Add sour cream and 1/4 cup sweetener and stir until smooth. Fold in whipped topping.

In the bottom of each glass, place 1 tablespoon graham cracker mix. Press down with spoon. Spoon 3 tablespoons cheese mixture on top of crumbs. Divide the cherries or among the glasses, placing them on top of the cream cheese layer. Add one more layer of cream cheese. Top each parfait with 1 tablespoon crumbs. Refrigerate till served.

Chocolate Chip Clouds

Servings: 30 • Serving Size: 1 cookie • Smart Points: 2

Calories: 53.7 • Fat: 2.2 g • Carb: 8.4 g • Fiber: 1.7 g • Protein: 1.1 g

Ingredients:

- 1/2 cup egg whites (room temperature) 1/8 tsp cream of tartar

- 1/2 cup sugar

- 1 tsp vanilla extract

- 2 tbsp unsweetened cocoa powder

- 1 cup chocolate chips

Directions:

Heat oven to 300°F. Cover cookie sheet with a nonstick silicone pad.

Using a mixer, beat the egg whites and cream of tartar until soft peaks form. Gradually add sugar a little at a time, then vanilla, beating well until you get stiff peaks, and the mixture is glossy.

Sift cocoa into egg whites, gently fold until combined.

Fold in chocolate chips. Drop mixture by heaping tablespoons onto cookie sheet.

Bake 34 to 40 minutes. Cool slightly then remove from cookie sheet. Cool completely on wire rack. Store covered, at room temperature. Do not make these on a rainy or humid day. Makes 30 to 32 cookies.

Coconut Tapioca Pudding with a Banana Kick

Serving size is about 1/2 cup Each serving = Smart Points = 5

164 calories; 6g fat; 5g saturated fat; 30g carbohydrates; 18g sugar; 2g protein; 2g fiber

Ingredients

- 1 Tbsp + 2 tsp small pearl tapioca

- 14 oz light, unsweetened coconut milk 1/2 tsp vanilla

- 1/4 C sugar

- 4 ripe bananas

Directions

Soak the tapioca in a small bowl of water for 1 hour to soften.

Combine the coconut milk, vanilla and sugar and cook over medium heat until the sugar

is dissolved. Stir constantly. Cool for 10 minutes. Peel 3 bananas, slice into small chunks. Drain the tapioca, and add with the bananas to the milk mixture. Stir while on a low simmer, until the mixture thickens. Refrigerate until cold, serve with slices of banana for garnish.

Double Chocolate Chip Biscotti

Servings: 24 • Size: 1 biscotti • Smart Points: 4

Calories: 100.9 • Fat: 2.9 g • Carb: 18.2 g • Fiber: 1.1 g • Protein: 1.9 g

Ingredients

- 1-2/3 cup all purpose flour

- 1/2 cup good quality unsweetened cocoa powder 1-1/2 tsp baking powder

- pinch of salt

- 3/4 cup superfine sugar (you can put sugar in food processor) 3/4 cup dark chocolate chips

- 2 large eggs

- 1 large egg white

Directions

Preheat oven to 375°. Line two cookie sheets with parchment paper.

Combine flour, cocoa powder, baking powder, chocolate chips, salt and sugar in a large bowl. Mix. Gradually add eggs and egg whites to the mixture and make a dough.

Divide the dough into three loaves. Place them on the lined baking sheets and bake 20 minutes. Cut into slices. Let cool.

Flourless Chocolate Cake

Servings: 8 • Serving Size: 1 cake • Smart Points: 6

Calories: 136 • Fat: 8 g • Sat Fat: 5 g • Protein: 3 g • Carb: 16 g • Fiber: 2 g Sugar: 11g • Sodium: 48 mg • Cholesterol: 23 mg

Ingredients:

- cooking spray
- 6 oz 60% Ghirardelli Chocolate 1/4 cup pumpkin puree
- 1 1/2 tbsp maple syrup
- 1 tsp vanilla extract
- 1 whole egg
- 3 egg whites
- 1/8 tsp kosher salt

Directions:

Preheat oven to 350°F. Grease 8 (4 oz) ramekins. Place on a large cooking sheet.

Melt chocolate in medium microwaveable bowl for 45 second intervals, until melted. Set aside to cool a few minutes.

Add the pumpkin puree, the vanilla, 1 whole egg, and maple syrup; mix well then fold into the melted chocolate.

Beat the egg whites until soft peaks form. Fold into the chocolate mixture. Add the salt. Spoon into the ramekins and bake 15 minutes, until the cakes rise. Serve warm.

<u>Key Lime Cheesecakes</u>

Makes 12 servings

Calories 140 : Carbohydrate 12g (Sugars 6g) : Total Fat 7g
(Sat Fat 4g) : Protein 7g : Fiber 0g : Cholesterol 35mg :
Sodium 270mg, Smart Point = 1

Ingredients

- ¾ cup graham cracker crumbs

- 2 tablespoons margarine or butter, melted

- 2 tablespoons plus ¾ cup no-calorie granulated
  sweetener, divided* 1 1/2 cups low-fat cottage
  cheese

- 8 ounces light tub-style cream cheese

- 3 tablespoons cornstarch

- 2 tablespoons Key lime juice

- Zest of 2 Key limes or 1 regular lime 1 teaspoon
  vanilla extract

- 1 large egg

- 1 large egg white

Directions

Preheat the oven to 325°F. Spray a 12-cup muffin tin.

Mix together the graham cracker crumbs, margarine, and 2 tablespoons of the sweetener until well combined.

Spoon a heaping tablespoon of this mixture into each muffin cup. Press gently. Blend the cottage cheese with the cream cheese, the remaining ¾ cup sweetener, the

cornstarch, lime juice, zest, and vanilla until creamy. Add the egg and the egg white and beat until just blended.

Place ¾ cup of cheesecake filling into each cup. Bake for 20 minutes, or until the cheesecakes are set, but centers wiggle a little. Cool and then chill at least 2 hours.

Low Fat Strawberry No-Bake Cheesecake

Servings: 8 • Serving Size: 1 slice • Smart Points: 6

Calories: 233.5 • Fat: 9.6 g • Protein: 3.1 g • Carb: 29.9 g • Fiber:1.5 g

Ingredients

- 8 oz Cool Whip Free
- 8 oz 1/3 less fat Philadelphia Cream Cheese

- 9 inch reduced fat Graham Cracker Crust 1/4 cup sugar

- 2 tsp vanilla extract

- 12-14 strawberries, hulled and halved lengthwise

Directions

Mix with a mixer the cream cheese, vanilla extract and sugar for a few minutes until fluffy. Add Cool Whip and mix until smooth. Spoon mixture into pie crust and chill for a few hours, until firm. Arrange strawberries in a circle on top and serve.

Mocha Mousse

2 Smart Points, 1 serving

Ingredients

- 1/2 cup part-skim ricotta cheese

- 1/2 teaspoon unsweetened cocoa powder 1/4 teaspoon vanilla extract

- 1 package sugar substitute

- 1 dash espresso powder

- 5 mini chocolate chips

Directions

Blend everything but the mini chocolate chips in a blender until creamy. Sprinkle with the chocolate chips and indulge.

Peanut Butter and Banana Ice Cream Recipe

1/2 cup is 129 calories, 4.3 g fat, 0.8 g saturated fat, 21.8 g carbohydrates, 11.3 g sugar, 3.5 g protein, 2.8 g fiber, 2 mg sodium, 4 Smart Points

Ingredients

- 3 very ripe bananas
- 2 tablespoons natural peanut butter (no sugar added)

Directions:

Slice bananas and place on a cookie sheet in a single layer. Freeze for 2 hours.

Take out of freezer and add peanut butter, placing both ingredients in a blender. Blend until smooth and creamy.

Skinny Strawberry Fool (with Cool Whip Free)

Servings: 6 • Serving Size: 3/4 cup • Smart Points 5 pts

Calories: 182 • Fat: 0.4 g • Protein: 5.9 g • Carb: 37.4 g • Fiber: 2.1 g Sodium: 73 mg

Ingredients:

For the strawberries:

- 1 1/2 lbs (3 1/2 cups) strawberries, washed, hulled, cut in half 1/3 cup Splenda

- pinch of salt

- 1/2 tsp grated lemon zest 1 1/2 tsp fresh lemon juice 8 oz Cool Whip Free

- 12 oz fat free Vanilla Chobani yogurt

Directions:

Combine the strawberries, Splenda, and salt in a bowl and stir until the strawberries are coated. Smash with a fork until half of the strawberries are smashed, but some medium sized chunks remain. Cook the strawberries over high heat, stirring occasionally, until bubbles form along the edge, about 5 minutes. Skim any foam with a spoon and discard. Add the lemon zest and lemon juice, stir to combine and bring to a full boil, 2 minutes more. Remove from heat, skim foam and discard. Cool to room temperature. Refrigerate 30 minutes.

When the strawberry sauce is cold, fold the whipped topping in a bowl along with the yogurt. Gently fold the strawberry sauce with the whipped cream to create pretty swirls and place in 6 glasses to serve.

Chapter 8: Recipes With Zero Smart Points!

Food recipes with zero smart points allow you to eat as much as you like without breaking the rules of the weight watchers program!

Best Tasting Weight Watchers Zero Points Vegetable Soup

Serves: 12, 1 cup = 1 serving, 0 Smart Points

Ingredients

- 2 medium garlic cloves), minced
- 1 medium onion(s), diced
- 2 medium carrots), diced
- 1 medium sweet red pepper(s), diced
- 1 medium stalk(s) celery, diced
- 2 medium zucchini, diced
- 1 medium yellow squash, diced
- 2 cups green cabbage, shredded
- 4 cups broccoli, small florets

- 2 tsp thyme, fresh, chopped

- 6 cups vegetable broth

- 2 Tbsp parsley, chopped ½ tsp table salt, or to taste

- ¼ tsp black pepper, or to taste

Instructions

Spray a large soup pot with cooking spray. Cook the onion, peppers, celery, and carrots for 7 minutes. Add the garlic and cook 2 minutes until softened. Next add in the zucchini, squash, and broccoli, then season with salt, pepper, and thyme, and cook about 5 minutes. Pour in the vegetable broth. Finally, mix the cabbage and parsley into the soup. Cover the pot and bring to a rapid boil, then simmer the ingredients at least 10 minutes. Let the soup cool, then blend in batches with a stand blender or an immersion blender. 1 serving is 1 cup.

Cabbage Soup With Zero Smart Points

Serves 1, SmartPoints 0

Ingredients

- 3 cup nonfat beef, vegetable, or chicken broth, beef is the best 2 garlic cloves, minced

- 1 tbsp tomato paste

- 2 cup cabbage, chopped 1/2 yellow onion

- 1/2 cup carrot, chopped 1/2 cup green beans

- 1/2 cup zucchini, chopped 1/2 tsp basil

- 1/2 tsp oregano 1 salt

- 1 black pepper

Directions

Spray pot cooking spray saute onions, carrots, and garlic for 5 minutes.

Add broth, Tomato paste, cabbage, green beans, basil, oregano and Salt & Pepper to taste. Simmer for 10 minutes, add the chopped zucchini and simmer 10 minutes more.

Slow Cooker Applesauce

yield: 6 (1/2 CUP) SERVINGS, SMARTPOINTS: 0 per serving

83 calories, 22 g carbs, 17 g sugars, 0 g fat, 0 g saturated fat, 1 g protein, 2 g fiber

Ingredients:

- 8 medium-large apples, peeled, cored and cut into wedges 1/4 cup water

- Cinnamon, to taste

Directions:

Place the apple pieces into your crock pot and cover with water. Cover and cook on low for 8 hours. Mash your apples to your desired texture. Add cinnamon starting with ½ tsp for taste. Cook for 15 more minutes to blend the flavors. Makes about 3 cups.

Weight Watchers Tortilla Soup with Zero Points!

0 SmartPoints, serving size 1 cup, servings 9,

51 calories per cup

Ingredients

- 1 cup onion, chopped

- 2 garlic cloves, chopped

- 3 green onions, chopped

- 2 (12 ounce) cans diced tomatoes

- 4 cups low-fat chicken broth 1/3 cup salsa

- 1/2 red pepper, chopped 1/2 green pepper, chopped 3 -4 celery ribs, chopped 1/3 cup fresh cilantro

- 1/2 teaspoon cumin1/2 teaspoon chili powder 1/2 teaspoon basil

- 4 tablespoons fat free sour cream

Directions

Simmer onions, garlic & green onions in chicken broth until tender. Place all the remaining ingredients into the pot, simmer for 30 minutes.

Chapter 9: Snacks With Only 1 Smart Point

Arctic Zero Creamy Pints

1/2 cup: 35 calories, 0g total fat (0g sat fat), 80 - 135mg sodium, 7g carbs, 2g fiber, 5g sugars, 3g protein -- Smart Points : 1

Ingredients

- Arctic Zero brand Frozen Dessert fresh fruit

Directions:

Scoop ½ cup of the frozen treat into a ramekin. Top with your favorite fruit.

BabyBel Snack Kabobs

1 piece: 50 calories, 3g total fat (2g sat fat), 160mg sodium, 0g carbs, 0g fiber, 0g sugars, 6g protein -- Smart Points : 1

Ingredients

- 1 small round of BabyBel light cheese, cut into 4 pieces 4 pieces of pineapple

- 4 pieces of honeydew melon

Directions

Place the BabyBel cheese on a skewer, followed by 2 pieces of fruit Continue until you have made a fruit kabob.

Bacon Cheeseburger Bites

yield: 24 PUFFS, Smart Points: 1 per puff, 4 for 4 puffs

44 calories, 3 g carbs, 0 g sugars, 2 g fat, 1 g saturated fat, 4 g protein, 0 g fiber

Ingredients:

- 6 oz raw 95% lean ground beef

- 1 tablespoon McCormick Hamburger seasoning

- 3 tablespoons finely chopped onion

- 1 clove garlic, minced

- 1 cup white whole wheat flour

- teaspoon baking powder 1/8 teaspoon salt

- 1/8 teaspoon crushed red pepper flakes

- 1 cup skim milk

- 1 large egg

- 4 oz reduced fat sharp cheddar cheese, shredded

- 3 tablespoons Hormel Real Bacon Bits

Directions:

Pre-heat the oven to 350. Lightly spray a 24 count mini muffin tin.

Cook the ground beef, add the hamburger seasoning and mix in. Cook until meat is browned. Add chopped onion and garlic and cook 2 more minutes.

Stir together flour, baking powder, salt and crushed red pepper. Add the milk and egg and whisk together. Add the ground beef mixture, cheese and bacon bits and stir well. Divide the batter evenly amongst the prepared mini muffin tin cups, about 1 T for each. Bake for 18-20 minutes.

Banana Pancake Bites

yield: 24 Pancake Bites, Smart Points: 1 per pancake bite

33 calories, 7 g carbs, 3 g sugars, 0 g fat, 0 g saturated fat, 1 g protein, 0 g fiber

Ingredients:

1 cup Bisquick Heart Smart Pancake & Baking Mix 2/3 cup skim milk

½ cup reduced calorie breakfast syrup

1 large ripe banana, chopped into small pieces

Directions:

Pre-heat the oven to 350. Lightly spray a 24 count mini muffin tin.

Stir together Bisquick mix, milk and syrup until smooth. Put 1 T of batter into each cup, top with banana pieces. Bake for 12-14 mins.

Bell Pepper Sweeties

Yields: 6 | Serving Size: 5 strips | Calories: 12 | Total Fat: 0 g | Saturated Fat: 0 g | Trans Fat: 0 g | Cholesterol: 0 | Carbohydrates: 3 g | Sodium: 4 mg | Dietary Fiber: 0 g | Sugars: 2 g | Protein: 0 g | SmartPoint: 1 |

Ingredients

- 2 red bell peppers, remove seeds, core and membrane

- 1 tablespoon pure maple syrup (less to taste)

Directions

Rinse peppers, slicing them to ½ inch strips. Dry well and drizzle with maple syrup. Make sure the peppers are well coated. Refrigerate for 2 hours in a covered bowl.

Preheat oven to 150F. Place the peppers on a wire rack covered with parchment paper in a single layer. Place the wire rack on a baking sheet, then place in the oven on the middle rack. Leave the oven door open 4 inches. Bake 10 hours, until the peppers are crispy. Store after cooling in a ziplock bag in the refrigerator.

Buffalo Tuna Boats

1 pouch: 70 calories, 0.5g total fat (0.5g sat fat), 620mg sodium, 0g carbs, 0g fiber, 0g sugars, 15g protein -- SmartPoints™ = 1

Ingredients

- 1 pouch Starkist Tuna Buffalo flavored
- 1 yellow bell pepper
- 1 tsp mayo

Directions:

Wash and seed the bell pepper, cutting it in half to make a boat. Mix the mayo (if you desire) and fill the boats with the tuna. Enjoy the crunchy snack.

Cheesecake Stuffed Strawberries

yield: 16 STRAWBERRIES, SMARTPOINTS: 1 per berry

35 calories, 5 g carbs, 3 g sugars, 2 g fat, 1 g saturated fat, 1 g protein, 0 g fiber

Ingredients:

- 1 lb fresh strawberries (this was about 16 large strawberries for me) 4 oz 1/3 less fat cream cheese, softened

- 1 cup powdered sugar

- teaspoon vanilla extract

- 1 full sized low fat graham cracker (one sheet of four little rectangles), crushed

Directions:

Cap the strawberries and throw away the greens. Hollow out each strawberry to leave a firm shell. In a mixing bowl, beat the cream cheese, powdered sugar and vanilla extract with an electric mixer until smooth. Fill each berry with the cheesecake mix. Dip each berry face down into the crumbs, to coat the cheesecake. Serve the same day.

Delightful Dill Dip

yield: 8 (1/4 CUP) SERVINGS, Smart Points: 1 per (1/4 cup) serving

39 calories, 5 g carbs, 3 g sugars, 0 g fat, 0 g saturated fat, 4 g protein, 0 g fiber

Ingredients:

- 1 cup fat free plain Greek yogurt

- 1 cup fat free sour cream

- 1.5 teaspoons dried parsley flakes

- 1 tablespoon dried chopped onion (also labeled as minced onion) 1 tablespoon dried dill weed

- 1 teaspoon seasoned salt ½ teaspoon garlic powder

Directions:

Combine all ingredients in a bowl and stir together until well combined. Cover and

refrigerate overnight or for at least 8 hours to allow flavors to combine.

Hard Boiled Egg Whites

3 large eggs' worth: 51 calories, <0.5g total fat (0g sat fat), 164mg sodium, 0.5g carbs, 0g fiber, 0.5g sugars, 10.5g protein -- Smart Points = 1

Ingredients:

- 3 large hard boiled eggs

- 1 tsp mayo

- 1 tsp mustard

- 2 tsp dill pickle relish

Directions:

Mix dill pickle relish, 1 tsp mayo, 1 tsp mustard and stuff the egg whites. Tastes just like deviled eggs.

Pimento Cheese Spread on the Skinny

Yields: 16 | Serving size: 2 tablespoons | Calories: 33 | Total Fat: 2 g | Saturated Fats: 1 g | Trans Fats: 0 g | Cholesterol: 4 mg | Sodium: 136 mg | Carbohydrates: 1 g | Dietary fiber: 0 g | Sugars: 1 g | Protein: 5 g | SmartPoints: 1 |

Ingredients

- 2 cups reduced fat cheddar cheese, shredded

- 1 green onion, diced

- 1 clove garlic, minced

- 8 ounces cream cheese, fat free (low-fat will work as well) 1/2 cup plain Greek yogurt, fat free

- 1 (4 ounce) jar diced pimentos, drained

- 1 small jalapeno pepper, seeded and minced 1/4 teaspoon black pepper

- Kosher or sea salt to taste 1/4 teaspoon cayenne pepper

Directions

Combine all ingredients and beat with an electric mixer until creamy. Refrigerate in a covered container until serving.

Peanut Butter Yogurt Dip

Serving size: 2 tablespoons | Calories: 40 | Saturated Fats: 1 gm | Trans Fats: 0 gm |

Cholesterol: 0 mg | Sodium: 6 mg | Carbohydrates: 2 gm | Dietary fiber: 0 gm | Sugars: 1 gm | Protein: 2 gm | SmartPoint: 1 |

Ingredients

- ½ cup Greek yogurt, fat free, plain

- ¼ cup natural peanut butter, crunchy recommended

Directions

Combine with a mixer, refrigerate until eating. Fantastic with zero point apples.

CHAPTER 10: SNACKS THAT ARE READY-MADE WITH ONLY 4 OR LESS SMART POINTS!

This is a list of snacks you can purchase while you are on the go, need something to eat, but don't want to blow your diet. All of these snacks have only 4 Smart Points.

1- Chex Mix, traditional (1/2 c.) Planter's cocktail peanuts (30) Planter's dry roasted peanuts (35)

2- Quaker Lower sugar maple and brown sugar (or apples and cinnamon) instant oatmeal (1 packet)

3- Quaker Chewy Chocolate chip granola bar (1) Sunchips, Multigrain snacks, original (15)

4- Post Honey Bunches of Oats with almonds cereal (3/4 c.)

5- One half of a Light English muffin with 1 tablespoon pasta sauce and 1 ounce low-fat mozzarella cheese baked until bubbly

6- A slice of reduced-calorie whole wheat bread toasted with 1 tablespoon peanut butter and banana slices

7- Mini Larabar, apple pie fruit and nut bar (1 bar) Healthy Choice Greek Dark Fudge Swirl Frozen Yogurt

8- 1/2 cup flake style imitation crab meat and 1 Tbsp. Lite Western dressing Vitalicious VitaTops, 100 calories, deep chocolate muffin top (1 vitatop) Kellogg's Special K Protein Greek yogurt and fruit granola snack bar (1 bar) Teddy graham graham snacks (10 pieces)

9- South Beach diet snack bar, whipped peanut butter (1 bar) Cheerios multi-grain cereal, dry (1 cup)

10- Popcorners Kettle popped corn chips (1 oz)

11- Wheat thins toasted chips, Great Plains Multigrain (13 chips)

Snacks With Only 3 Smart Points

1- Keebler pretzel thins (8)

2- Keebler Club crackers, minis, multigrain (24) Apple slices with 1 tablespoon peanut butter

3- Two stalks of celery with 1 tablespoon peanut butter A cup of broth based vegetable soup

4- Three ounces turkey and sliced tomato on 1 slice whole-wheat bread Eight baked low-fat tortilla chips and 2 Tbsp. fat free black bean dip Emerald Cocoa roast dark chocolate almonds, 100 calorie pack (1 pack) Emerald Natural walnuts and almonds, 100 calorie pack (1 pack)

5- 2 oz. ham in a Ole High fiber low carb tortilla wrap 3 oz. shrimp with 2 Tbsp. cocktail sauce

6- 1 brown rice cake with 2 tsp. peanut butter and strawberries Pringles Stix honey butter flavored snack sticks (1 pack) Sun-Maid Mini-snacks natural California raisins (1 box) Kashi TLC snack crackers,

Original 7 grain (12 crackers) Mini Wheats Frosted cereal, bite size, dry (1/2 cup)

Snacks With Only 2 Smart Points

1- Dannon Activia light nonfat yogurt, strawberry (1 container) Pop Secret Kettle corn popcorn (1 cup)

2- One-half cup sliced or baby carrots and 2 tablespoons hummus hard-boiled egg (1)

3- Wheat thins whole grain crackers (8)

4- Sensible portions garden veggie straws with sea salt (22 straws) Pistachios, in shells (22)

5- Carrots with 2 Tbsp. reduced fat ranch dressing

6- Sargento Light Mozzarella Cheese stick wrapped in 2 oz. sliced turkey Tri-color pepper strips, 9 baked low-fat tortilla chips and fat-free salsa 1 scrambled egg with fat-free salsa

7- 1 pear, 1 Weight Watcher string cheese and 7
    almonds Thick sliced carrots dipped in 3 Tbsp.
    guacamole

8- 3 cups light microwave popcorn

9- Goldfish snack crackers, baked cheddar (30 pieces)
    Fit & Active rice cakes (8 mini cakes)

10- Crispix cereal, dry (1/2 cup) Butterball turkey bacon
    (5 slices)

Snacks With Only 1 Smart Point

1- Almonds (7)

2- Rold Gold Pretzel sticks (20)

3- One-half cup nonfat cottage cheese and a piece of
    fruit Butter flavored popcorn (1 cup)

4- grapes and 1 oz. low-fat cubed Swiss cheese 1 /4 cup light vanilla yogurt and blueberries

5- 1 Tbsp. low-fat cream cheese in 4 small pieces celery drizzled with hot sauce 1/4 c. fat-free black bean dip with fresh veggies

6- A medium apple or pear with 1 stick of Sargento Light mozzarella string cheese Mini Babybel Light semisoft cheese (1) and fruit

7- One Laughing Cow Light Garlic & Herb wedge spread on cucumber slices 3 slices white meat turkey rolled in 3 lettuce leaves

8- 1 pretzel rod

9- Boca Original vegan veggie burger (1 burger)

10- Old Wisconsin Snack sticks, turkey sausage (1 stick)

11- A bowl of blueberries and 2 Tbsp. lite whipped topping

CONCLUSION

Thank you again for downloading this book!

I hope this book was able to help you to find delicious Weight Watcher recipes to cook and enjoy.

Now that you have enticing recipes and a known method of losing weight, we wish you success in your journey.

If you have enjoyed this book, please make a comment on Amazon.

Good luck!

<u>One Last Thing For You!</u>

To check out more of Sarah's books, visit her author page on Amazon.com by searching "Sarah Lynch"

About The Author

Sarah Lynch earned her M.D. from Baylor College of Medicine and her ph.D. from John Hopkins University, along with a B.A. from the University of Chicago, where she studied Nutrition Science.

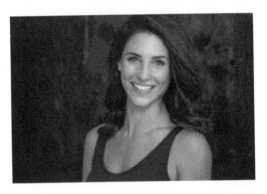

Sarah is a world renowned Certified Holistic Life Coach with 7 years experience in practice and coaching the Holistic lifestyle approach. Her specialties revolve around diet/nutrition, spirituality, emotional brain training and much more. As a holistic coach her work is directed towards the achievement of all her clients goals through physical, mind and spiritual training.

Printed in Poland
by Amazon Fulfillment
Poland Sp. z o.o., Wrocław